# Essential Oils: Discover the Drug-Free, Safe & Inexpensive Way to Combat Anxiety & Stress with 20 DIY Recipes

By Lauren Marshall

**Medical Disclaimer**

This book is not intended as a substitute for the medical advice of physicians. The reader should regularly consult a physician in matters relating to his/her health and particularly with respect to any symptoms that may require diagnosis or medical attention. Any recommendations given in this book are not a substitute for medical advice.

# Contents


**Essential Oils: Discover the Drug-Free, Safe & Inexpensive Way to Combat Anxiety & Stress with 20 DIY Recipes**........ 1

Contents................................................................4

Introduction............................................................ 5

An Overview of Essential Oils...............................13

Some Essential Oil Terminology...........................18

Essential Oils Vs Fragrance Oils and Perfumes.................... 25

Essential Oils Throughout History...........................31

Aromatherapy........................................... 44

The Most Popular Essential Oils...........................51

Quick Ailment Reference Guide...........................79

Creating Your Own Essential Oil Blends - DIY Recipes.........85

Conclusion................................................. 103

Other books by Lauren Marshall...........................107

# Introduction

As little as a few decades ago, essential oils were not very popular in mainstream western culture. Although many different cultures throughout history have utilized essential oils for medicinal and spiritual purposes, much of the knowledge regarding their value was lost. Instead, the subject was deemed a new-age fad, relegated to the same territory as astrology, fortune telling and reading auras. It was not until the end of the twenty-first century that we began to see a renewed interest in the subject. Today, aromatherapy is a reputable subject for practice and study, and essential oils are readily available. You can find them not only in specialty stores geared towards natural healing, but also in major drugstore and on line as well!

It may be difficult for those who are unfamiliar with the subject to believe that essential oils and aromatherapy actual have any true healing properties. Yet, even the most skeptical critic cannot deny the how influential our sense of smell is. Certain smells can trigger memories better than any of our other senses, and these smells also have a marked effect on our mood and state of mind. For example, many people associate the smell of fresh cut grass with summertime. Exposure to the scent triggers receptors in the brain that increase happiness and promote a relaxed, carefree feeling, much as we used to experience during the long warm days of our childhood. Likewise, certain smells may carry negative connotations for certain people. As an example, the smell of gasoline may trigger anxiety and even outright panic in people who have been involved in car accidents.

It is not only the way that smells affect our mood and mental state that makes aromatherapy such an interesting discipline. Certain essential oils also carry some very valid healing qualities. Citrus oils are remarkably stimulating and can assist with elevating energy levels while also increasing the immune system. Tea tree oil is excellent for discouraging ticks and biting insects, while peppermint oil discourages mice and spiders from taking up residence in an area. Lavender oil has been proven to drastically reduce the intensity of migraine headaches, while chamomile oil is wonderful for combatting insomnia and night terrors.

Essential oils are also utilized in many different beauty products. For example, even the most exclusive, pricy designer perfumes are basically composed of one or more essential oils which have been diluted with water. Likewise, a huge amount of personal care items ranging from very expensive to remarkably cheap use essential oils for fragrance and therapeutic benefits. These include soaps, lotions, shampoos, bath bombs, etc. Some companies elect to use fragrance oils instead of essential oils, which means the consumer receives the aromatic smell of the plant but reaps none of the healing benefits.

Historically, essential oils were used out of sheer practicality as well as for their value in medicine, ceremony and spiritual areas. In the days before we had access to flush toilets, running water, refrigeration and other modern conveniences, living conditions were often less than sanitary. Human waste was collected in chamber pots and tossed out into the street, and as there was no garbage man who made the rounds weekly, rotting produce and other waste was often left in the streets to fester. In some areas that were particularly hard hit with plague and other diseases, corpses could be left in piles before they were able to be buried in a mass grave or burned. As one might expect, the result was a powerfully unpleasant smell that permeated the air, as well as an infestation of fleas, rats and other pests running rampant, leading to prime conditions for the farther spread of disease.

Essential oils were not only valued for their ability to cover up the worst of the horrific smell, some were also used for their anti-septic and anti-biotic qualities, as well as for their ability to keep disease spreading pests at bay.

In modern times, we utilize essential oils for cosmetic reasons as well as for the benefits they provide for the mind, body and soul. While essential oils are readily available and anyone can choose to purchase and work with them, it is very important to have a basic working knowledge as to what essential oils are, and what they can and cannot do before beginning to use them. There are definite risks and potentially negative side effects which can occur if you carelessly experiment without knowing what you are doing. As we will discuss more in depth later on, the essential oil market is not very well regulated. In fact, the Food and Drug Administration does not even have a precise definition for essential oils, instead treating them exactly the same as the plant source they came from. The FDA also does not distinguish between essential oils and fragrance oils, so it is very important to know exactly what you are looking for and read the labels before making a purchase. The way that companies advertise is not heavily regulated either. This means that manufacturers can put labels on their bottles which sound appealing and make them stand out from other selections, yet in reality, the terms they use don't really mean anything at all.

The aim of this book is to provide the reader with a basic introduction to essential oils and aromatherapy. Here, you will learn about the benefits as well as the potential risks associated with certain oils, as well as exploring the most popular oils available for purchase today. You will even learn how to create your own essential oil blends to tailor them to your exact need, as well as receiving instruction on how to properly store them for maximum longevity.

Essential oils are wonderful to experiment with once you know what you are doing, so be sure to take the time to educate yourself about each and every oil you choose to utilize. This book will provide you with a basic overview, yet it is necessary to keep in mind that there may be potential risks associated with particular oils that are not specifically covered here. In regards to children and animals, it is always better to be safe than sorry and store the essential oils well out of reach. If your are pregnant or nursing, be sure to consult with your doctor before using any kind of essential oil internally, externally or aromatically.

# An Overview of Essential Oils

So what exactly are essential oils? This is a question that can be very confusing for someone who is just beginning to explore the subject, as there is no precise definition. The best way to describe an essential oil is to say that it is a super-concentrated form of a specific plant. Each and every plant contains natural oils within it. These natural oils are in place to create a natural barrier against potential predators and diseases. Because these oils protect the plant, they are necessary, or essential to the vitality of the plant's life. As long the oils are in place, the plant generally remains healthy and unharmed. These oils are found in the plant's blossoms, leaves, bark, resin and roots, and they constitute the major component of essential oils.

When you pick a lavender blossom, you can certainly inhale the scent and derive some of the plant's aromatic gifts. However, a small bottle of lavender essential oil is the end the result of a significant amount of the blossoms which have been condensed into a singular, powerful oil. In the process of becoming an essential oil, everything that is not therapeutic has been removed from the lavender, leaving you only with the parts that have medicinal and spiritual value. Essential oils are far more potent than a plant in its natural form. In fact, many times, a singular drop is enough to produce results! Peppermint oil is another good example. While you can certainly gather fresh or dried peppermint leaves and leave them in the corners of your home to discourage mice and spiders, you can achieve even better results with just a drop or two of the essential oil on a cotton ball!

When you look at a cedar tree, it is difficult to understand how that giant tree could possibly wind up in a small bottle that can be carried around in the pocket. The process of extracting essential oils from the raw plants is something that typically occurs via two different methods – steam distillation and mechanical expression.

Steam distillations uses super-heated steam to release the oils from their protective sacs within the plant. The heat from the steam forces its way through the tiny pores in the plant and collects the oils with it as it passes through. The steam turns into water in a condensation chamber, and the oils rise to the top of the mixture, allowing for easy collection.

Mechanical expression, on the other hand, uses gravity rather than heat for extraction. Essential oils that are obtained via mechanical expression rather than steam distillation may also be referred to as cold pressed. Instead of collection the oils via the use of extreme temperatures, they are instead literally pressed out of the plant via the use of tremendous force and gravitational pull.

The vast majority of essential oils you can find available for purchase are obtained via steam distillation. While this is by far the more common of the two extraction methods, the exception to the rule is in regards to essential oils which are obtained from citrus fruit. Wild orange, grapefruit, lemon and lime oils are all derived via mechanical expression, as the oil comes from applying force to the rind rather than any part of the plant that could be easily distilled.

# Some Essential Oil Terminology

Particularly when you are just beginning to learn about and work with essential oils, choosing the right ones can be confusing at best and completely overwhelming at worst. There are a number of different brands and varieties to choose from, and it is very important to be aware that some of these companies will intentionally try to market their essential oils with clever wording and flashy labels to make their product appear to be superior to the competition.

In the process of exploring your choices, you may come across certain bottles of essential oils which carry a label which reads "therapeutic grade."

Although the terminology sounds good and may even initially convince you that this particular oil choice is stronger, purer or more valuable for health benefits and aromatherapy purposes, the reality is that the therapeutic grade label means absolutely nothing. This is certainly not to say that the essential oil in question is inferior to other products, it just means that it is not necessarily any better either.

There is no precise or defined set of guidelines in place that deals with regulating different grades and qualities of essential oils. In fact, there is very little regulation in place regarding essential oils in general, as the FDA labels them both a cosmetic and a drug and makes decisions on a case by case basis. As there is no true regulation, the term therapeutic grade is rendered null and void, as any company can elect to use that wording, regardless of their qualifications. It is simply a label that is freely put on the bottle to make the product appear more attractive to the customer rather than a term that carries any kind of true significance.

You will also come across essential oils that are labeled pure vs blended. Here, those two terms definitely do mean two separate and distinct products, and the difference is exactly what it sounds like. An essential oil that is labeled one hundred percent pure means that that bottle of oil contains the oils of only one plant species, while a blend is made up of anywhere from one to many different essential oils. For example, if you are exploring essential oils to assist with a lack of energy, you may elect to purchase a bottle of one essential oil that carries a strong reputation for increasing vitality, such as peppermint, lemon or eucalyptus. However, you may also choose to purchase a pre-blended bottle of oil that contains all three of these individual oils which is specifically geared towards combatting lethargy.

So, is it better to work with pure essential oils, or blended oils? As with everything, there are distinct advantages and setbacks associated with both.

Pure oils are nice to work with because you know exactly what you are getting every time. If you are electing to utilize an essential oil for a particular need, it is important to use a product that contains that oil and that oil only. For example, tea tree oil is very beneficial for the skin, and has the ability to repel insects and ticks. This makes tea tree oil an ideal choice for hikers and those who spend a lot of time outdoors.

Pure tea tree oil can be applied to the skin and generally tolerated without any major irritation, however, if you were to apply a blend of tea tree and lemon to your skin, the risks of obtaining a severe sunburn are substantial, as the addition of lemon oil results in heightened photosensitivity.

Anyone who crafts their own essential oil blends must begin with pure oils as a basic stepping stone. If you buy a bottle of pure lavender oil, you can build your own blends precisely to achieve the results you want, whereas if you are trying to work with a lavender blend, there are variables in your recipe that you may be unaware of.  Unless you have created the blended oil yourself, it is virtually impossible to be confident of the exact contents.

Blended oils certainly have their advantages as well.  While some people may take great delight in concocting their own special blends, others may be interested in utilizing essential oils, but do not have the time or finances to explore each oil individually.  Instead of purchasing three or four separate oils and blending them together in precise proportions, it is far more convenient to buy one professionally preblended oil that is specifically geared towards a specific purpose, such as alleviating anxiety or promoting focus and concentration.  Those with a busy, on-the-go lifestyle are particularly drawn to essential oil blends, as they can simply place a few drops of one oil into their diffuser and walk away rather than concocting a specialized formula each day.

Aside from convenience, blended oils tend to have the financial edge. Pure essential oils require a large number of raw plant material to produce a small amount of oil. The extraction process can be quite tedious and long, which is why some essential oils, such as neroli and tuberose are extremely expensive in their pure form yet become significantly more affordable when added to a blend.

# Essential Oils Vs Fragrance Oils and Perfumes

It can be very confusing to try and distinguish the key difference essential oils and fragrance oils. While some may presume that essential oils are what give a scented candle or air freshener its appealing smell, this is not always true. Oftentimes, these products obtain their scent from synthetic fragrance oils rather than essential oils, which means that the aroma is created in a laboratory rather than in nature. This is the primary difference between essential oils and fragrance oils – one is one hundred percent natural, while the other is not. As a result, the scent you will obtain from product which incorporates lavender fragrance oil may smell exactly the same as products which utilize pure lavender oil, yet in contrast to the pure form, the synthetic version will supply zero health or therapeutic benefits.  A bar of soap containing actual lavender oil will not only soften the skin and sooth sunburn, it will contribute a sense of tranquility to the bathing process as well. While lavender soaps scented with synthetic fragrance oils may still provide the appealing smell, the therapeutic benefits do not exist.

Perfumes are created in a laboratory while essential oils are created by mother nature. Synthetic perfume oils serve one purpose, and one purpose only. This is to create a smell which appealing to the human nose. Some designer labels demand upwards of hundreds of dollars for a small bottle of their signature perfume, yet in making this purchase, the customer is paying for sheer smell alone. There are absolutely zero

therapeutic benefits associated with even the priciest,

most exclusive synthetic fragrance. Even though these

companies may advertise that they contain beneficial

scents, such as jasmine, lavender or ylang-ylang, these

scents are not derived from a natural source, meaning

they are not the same.

Not only do synthetic perfume oils tend to be

far more expensive than essential oil blends with a

similar fragrance, the perfume oil scent is diluted with

water or alcohol. Not only does this mean that the

fragrance will evaporate from the skin in much less

time, it also can leave the skin dried out and irritated

from the alcohol.

Essential oils can be applied to the pulse points of the body, such as the inner wrists, inside of the knees and along the throat one time per day, and the scent will continue to be noticeable. Because the oil is super-concentrated rather than diluted, it is long lasting. This means that you not only have to apply your fragrance less often, it means that you use less product, which ultimately saves on money.

Some people have respiratory issues and/or allergies that result in an extreme adverse reaction to synthetic perfume oils. These same individuals are also usually able to tolerate using essential oils, as the natural compounds are not as irritating to the lungs as the synthetic product. This is particularly true in the case of scented candles, air fresheners and other products that rely upon synthetic perfume oils rather than essential oils for fragrance. Not only do these products not carry any therapeutic benefits, even though their label may imply otherwise, they may actually cause harm, as they are essentially diffusing chemicals throughout the area they are used in.

It does bear mentioning that many essential oils are extremely irritating to the skin when applied directly out of the bottle. It is therefore always necessary to utilize a good, quality carrier oil (more on this later) to help create a boundary between the essential oil and the skin. It is also a good idea to do your research beforehand regarding any oil you plan on using. Some essential oils, such as orange, lemon and cinnamon are extremely reactive to sunlight, so you definitely don't want to be wearing them if you're planning on spending the day at the beach or hitting up the tanning bed. As a general precaution, it is always wise to do an allergy/irritant spot test on a very small area of skin before working with the oil.

# Essential Oils Throughout History

**China:** Nature and the natural world has always figured heavily into traditional Chinese medicine; therefore, it comes as no surprise that China is currently one of the biggest exporters of essential oils in the entire world! Chinese medicine uses essential oils for therapeutic ailments. Traditionally, Chinese aromatherapy involves the combination of three separate fragrances, which serve as a top, base and middle note. The top, or high note is intended to disappear quickly, while the middle notes last around eight hours. The base note, however, is the most enduring, in some cases lasting up to two days! Three separate oils may be combined to combat a psychological, spiritual or physical ailment, or simply one may be used, depending upon the situation. For example, a simple top note of something citrus, such as lemon or orange may be all that is needed to restore vitality, while those with chronic fatigue may require the three-fold blend, consisting of a citrus top note and longer acting middle and base notes.

In Chinese culture, any essential oil is believed to be infused with the essence or raw life force of the plant it came from. This essence is called *jing*, and it is a very powerful component in achieving balance between the heart, mind, body and soul as well as for healing a variety of physical and mental ailments. Essential oils are frequently used in conjunction with acupuncture, another ancient form of Chinese medicine that involves stimulating various areas of the body via the insertion of tiny, thin needles.

**Egypt:** Research shows that essential oils were being used in Egypt as early as 4500 BC! In fact, during ancient Egypt's heyday, you had to be a priest or someone of tremendous spiritual significance in order to work firsthand with essential oils. These oils were considered to be gifts from the gods, and they were therefore too valuable and too sacred to be entrusted in the hands of everyday people. Thus, they were given to those who were seen as being closet to the Gods. The priests were educated in the subject and could distribute the oils accordingly to those who they determined were in need of them, yet they alone had the privilege and/or knowledge of mixing and storing the oils.

The ancient Egyptians were a deeply spiritual culture. They attributed magical qualities to everything from certain animals, such as cats and crocodiles to various plants that were used for ceremonial purposes as well as healing. The ancient Egyptians are responsible for the creation of Kyphi, a blend of over sixteen essential oils that was used in the temples for its extreme spiritual value. Various deities, such as Bastet, Ra and Osiris had their own sacred essential oil blends which were used in ceremony to invoke their favor by anointing their statues. Each Pharo was considered to be an embodiment of the divine, thus they all had their own select blends of oils which were specifically created for them by the priests. These oils were used for many different purposes, depending upon the need at the time. Some would use their oil blend to anoint their weapons before going into battle with the enemy, while others would sprinkle the oil upon their bedsheets to improve their virility and to encourage healthy heirs.

The benefits of essential oils were not only limited to the priests and pharos, however. Cleopatra herself was said to be a huge fan of essential oils from a very young age. She reportedly had a number of blends crafted for her which she regularly used for everything from enhancing her legendary beauty to seducing potential suitors to granting protection from the evil eye.

**Greek/Roman:** Ancient Greek/Roman culture heavily incorporated essential oils into their everyday lives as well as utilizing them for ceremonial and other spiritual purposes.  Certain blends were used to anoint and perfume the body to grant protection and increase bravery before going into battle, while other oils were incorporated into massages and baths to promote relaxation and to increase morale.

Hippocrates was an ancient Greek physician who lived from 460 – 370 BC. If you're not already familiar with his work, he was often referred to as the Father of Modern Medicine, each and every physician must agree to abide by the Hippocratic Oath before commencing practice, meaning that they agree to adhere to a basic code of ethical conduct when they agree to take on the title of doctor. Hippocrates was a strong advocate for aromatherapy or using essential oils for a therapeutic purpose. In order to live a long, healthy live, he believed that every person should indulge daily in an aromatic bath followed by a rigorous massage which also incorporated essential oils.

It is believed that the Greeks were one of the first cultures to begin documenting written knowledge of essential oils, though most of this knowledge was taken from Egyptian culture.

**India:** The form of healing that was practiced in ancient India is typically referred to as Ayurveda. Ayurvedic medicine is one of the oldest documented medicinal systems in the entire world, originating sometime well over three thousand years ago!  The system is centered around the concept of chakras, which are particular areas in the body where energy tends to concentrate. Different essential oils are known to have an effect on different chakras, making them a valuable addition to reiki, meditation and other practices which rely upon balancing the energy of a person's chakras.

- **The Root Chakra:** Located at the base of the spine, this is the chakra that rules over our basic sense of security and belonging in the world. Root chakra work responds to essential oils that are grounding and earth-based in nature, such as patchouli or myrrh.

- **The Sacral Chakra:** Located just below the belly button, this is the chakra that rules over our sense of sexuality, sensuality, passion and creativity. The sacral chakra responds to essential oils that have an aphrodisiac, libido enhancing quality, such as ylang-ylang and sandalwood.

- **The Solar Plexus Chakra:** This is the warrior chakra, the part of our body that determines energy, self-esteem and confidence in our interactions with the world. Working with this chakra requires the ability to honest evaluate oneself, as one may need more cooling or heating oils, depending upon the state of being. For example, if you are a person who tend to have difficulty speaking up for yourself, you may want to concentrate on more stimulating, fiery oils such as cinnamon or black pepper while those who have trouble keeping their tempers in check may benefit from a more soothing, cooling oil such as wintergreen or eucalyptus. Both oils stimulate the chakra, just in a different way.

- **The Heart Chakra:** Located at the heart, this is the center of emotion in the body. Stimulating the heart chakra promotes romance and a relief from anxiety and depression, while the solar plexus chakra regulates the sexual aspects of a relationship. The heart chakra is what binds us to the people we love, as well as that which gives us the strength to endure uncomfortable emotions, such as fear and depression. The heart chakra is affected by essential oils which promote romance and an overall sense of well-being, such as rose and geranium.

- **The Throat Chakra:** The throat chakra, as one would expect, is located in the center of the throat. This chakra rules over our ability to express ourselves and may require attention anytime we feel as though we are afraid to speak up for ourselves, or on the other end of the spectrum, anytime we find ourselves being untruthful or intentionally manipulating others with our words. Healthwise, this is the chakra that has a direct effect on the respiratory system, so those who smoke or experience allergies may find themselves to be particularly benefitted by working with essential oils geared towards this area. The most common essential oils for the throat chakra are mentholated in nature, meaning that peppermint, eucalyptus, wintergreen, spearmint, etc. are often the top choices.

- **The Third Eye Chakra:** Located in the center of the forehead, the third eye chakra is associated with clairvoyance and the ability to perceive and move through the boundaries between our world and spiritual realms. Essential oils associated with the third eye chakra, such as juniper, clary sage and heliotrope are meant to increase our receptivity to spiritual energies while removing psychic and mental blockages. The third eye chakra is a particularly beneficial spot for treating restlessness, attention deficient disorder or even the simple inability to focus and concentrate.

- **The Crown Chakra:** Located at the very top of the head, the crown chakra is our gateway to heaven, the communication point between us on earth and the divine realm. This is the chakra that controls our sense of spirituality as well as that which

assists us with delving into mysterious realms,

such as clairvoyance, etc. The essential oils which

are associated with the crown chakra are those

that establish a kind of hot-line between our realm

and the otherworld, such as frankincense and

elemi.

# Aromatherapy

The National Association for Holistic Aromatherapy defines aromatherapy as an "art and science of utilizing naturally extracted aromatic essences from plants to balance, harmonize and promote the health of mind, body and spirit." Simply put, the aromatherapy is the practice of using essential oils to alter ones physical, mental or emotional state of mind.

Before we get into depth about different essential oils and their individual uses, it is important to understand how essential oils are used in aromatherapy in the first place. There are three primary methods of delivering essential oils to the body. These include inhalation, topical absorption and internal ingestion.

Internal ingestion is by far the most controversial and risky method of using essential oils. While some people think nothing of putting a drop of lemon oil in their daily water bottle, it is important to be aware that very few essential oils have actually been deemed safe for internal use. The bottom line is that the research simply isn't there, therefore the long-term risks are unknown. Unless it is absolutely known to be safe, internal use of essential oils is discouraged, particularly in the cases of children or nursing and/or pregnant women. While it is certainly possible for experts to reap the internal benefits of consuming essential oils, there are far less risky and invasive methods that deliver substantial results, as we will discuss below.

The two most common methods of utilizing essential oils lies in topical or aromatic use. Topical use means that the essential oil is applied to the skin, while aromatic use means that the scent is inhaled via a diffuser or simply worn as a perfume for its aromatic benefits.

Many essential oils are beneficial to the skin in a number of ways. Tea Tree oil, for example, can be applied directly to the skin to ward against ticks, mosquitoes, black flies as well as guarding against funguses like athlete's foot and other contagious conditions. Lavender is particularly soothing to the skin and acts as a natural anti-microbial and demulcent, working to regenerate damaged skin cells and minimizing damage from scalds, burns and overexposure to the sun.

Other essential oils have beneficial topical properties, yet they are too powerful in their concentrated form to be applied directly to the skin. This is where the concept of a carrier oil comes into play. Selecting a good quality carrier oil is essential in the practice of aromatherapy, as the carrier oil is what creates a protective boundary between the concentrated essential oil and one's bare skin. Oftentimes, the most popular carrier oils, such as coconut, jojoba, almond, olive and/or Argon oil carry skin-enhancing benefits by themselves as well, including demulcent and emollient properties.

A number of essential oils are highly valued for their ability to repel insects and ticks. Many of these, such as tea tree, peppermint, juniper and eucalyptus can be freely applied to the skin as long as they are diluted in water first. While more information can be found in the essential oil recipe section, a general rule of thumb is to add anywhere from 10 – 20 drops of essential oil to two tablespoons of carrier oil. Likewise, a lightweight, emergency bug spray that is far gentler for children involves a simple 10 drops of essential oil combined with two cups of water and sprayed on exposed areas of the skin as well as on clothing.

By far, the most popular method of using essential oils in aromatherapy is, as one would expect, aromatically. This means that you are directly inhaling the fragrance from the essential oil in order to access its therapeutic and/or spiritual properties.  The most common method of delivering essential oils in an aromatherapeutic environment is via a diffuser. Diffusers are an all-natural counterpart to scented candles, and they carry far more health benefits and less risks with them as well.

Some diffusers are made out of rods dipped in essential oil which travels up the rod and diffuses the scent throughout the room, though the most common and potent diffusers are made out of a small glass bowl that is filled with water and five drops of a particular essential oil before being placed above a burning tea light candle. The heat from the candle heats the water and oil, diffusing the scent throughout the area. Other methods include adding drops of oil to bath water or incorporating them into a massage.

While aromatic use is by far the safest way to work with essential oils, it is still not entirely without its risks.  Particularly if you are nursing or pregnant, be sure to consult your doctor before using essential oils in any form and keep them well out of the reach of children and animals.

# The Most Popular Essential Oils

1. **Angelica:** Angelica oil is derived via steam distillation of the seeds. It is a wonderful essential oil for increasing levels of energy, concentration and overall alertness. Diffuse a few drops of the oil throughout a room while studying or reading for increased clarity and focus, as well as for an overall boost in creativity and inspiration!

Angelica oil is also wonderful for combatting feelings of lethargy and a lack of energy associated with depression and/or anxiety. It can also assist with relieving respiratory issues as well as with lessening the severity and frequency of migraine headaches.

Pregnant and/or nursing women should avoid angelica oil in all forms, as it can be toxic to the baby.

2.  **Basil:** Basil oil is associated with drawing good luck and prosperity to a home. A few drops of oil diffused throughout an area will help to increase money flow, while inhaling the oil on a regular basis is also believed to stimulate the mood, increase energy levels and promote an overall sense of joy.

Basil oil is also wonderful for alleviating migraine headaches as well as for encouraging the appetite. It is an effective anti-emetic as well, meaning that it can soothe nausea and upset stomachs.

Basil oil should never be used internally, as it can be toxic and even fatal in the wrong doses.

3.  **Bergamot:** Generally obtained via mechanical expression, bergamot promotes a general sense of well-being, joyfulness and child-like gratitude for the moment at hand. This makes it valuable essential oil for those battling depression and anxiety, as well as for anyone with a generalized sense of overwhelming stress.

On a physical level, bergamot oil has helped with liver and spleen ailments, as well as encouraging the appetite.

It is however, very important to be aware that bergamot oil is very photosensitive. This means that is can cause irritation to the skin by itself if it is applied with no carrier oil, yet even when the best precautions are taken, it does not react well with direct sunlight. If you are planning on spending time in the sunshine, avoid applying bergamot oil to the skin for at least

twenty-four hours before exposure, as severe burns

and even blistering can result!

4.  **Cedar:** Cedar bark was burned by Native
Americans for its ability to purify the spirit and to
promote divine protection, and it is used for much
the same purposes in modern aromatherapy.
Cedar is a scent that is considered to be
particularly sacred to the Gods, thus its aroma is
believed to ward against all kinds of evil, including
repelling diseases and residual negative energy.
Adding a few drops of cedar oil to the corners of a
home will cleanse the area of any harmful energies
that may be lurking, making this a particularly
powerful oil for anyone in need of psychic
protection. Cedar oil is also wonderful for
improving mental clarity along with promoting
wisdom and spiritual awareness.

Medicinally, cedar is a wonderful remedy for mild respirator ailments, such as bronchitis or seasonal allergies.

Cedar oil is best used aromatically. It can be toxic in some individuals even when ingested in small doses, and it is very irritating to the skin when used topically. Pregnant women should avoid all forms of use of cedar oil.

5.  **Chamomile:** Obtained from the steam distillation of the blossoms, chamomile is well-known for its sedative, calming qualities. The oil can be diffused throughout a room to promote restfulness and to guard against nightmares, while applying it topically works to repel insects. According to some folk legends, chamomile oil is considered very lucky, and can attract wealth and good fortune to

anyone who anoints themselves with the oil.

Washing your hands in a cup of water that has been mixed with ten drops of chamomile oil is said to encourage monetary flow and professional success, while the oil itself can be used to combat acne, bruising and other skin ailments.

It is interesting to note that those who experience an allergic reaction to ragweed tend to have adverse reactions to using chamomile oil aromatically, so be sure to educate yourself about the potential risks before use. Chamomile oil is not safe for internal use, and any form of ingestion should be avoided unless you are an expert.

6.  **Cinnamon:** Cinnamon oil is a very powerful, active essential oil with a number of potent properties. First, it is invigorating, serving to increase alertness and levels of energy. It is considered a very lucky oil as well, working to draw money and prosperity towards anyone who works with the scent. Cinnamon oil not only boosts creativity and overall stamina, it is extremely useful in elevating passion on all levels. This means that it not only increases the libido and draws romantic energy, it can also assist with improving levels of self-confidence and combatting shyness, indifference and/or introversion.  Cinnamon oil is very active, which means that it helps to provide speed and intensity to any other oil it is coupled with. This makes it a

very potent addition to essential oil blends which

are intended to draw love or money.

On a physical level, cinnamon oil helps to strengthen

the immune system, and stimulates circulation.


7.   **Eucalyptus:** Eucalyptus oil has a powerful,

distinctive odor. It is a wonderful oil for students,

as it promotes concentration and increases mental

clarity. A few drops of eucalyptus oil diffused

throughout a room while studying helps with

retaining information, as well as with eliminating

outside distractions.

Medicinally, eucalyptus oil is a highly effective

respiratory aid. It can also be used as a febrifuge,

meaning it can combat fevers by lowering the body

temperature when the oil is applied to the chest area.

Eucalyptus oil has also shown to be an effective remedy against migraine headaches.

It is important to note that eucalyptus oil should not be used in any form by those with epilepsy or other convulsive disorders, as it can trigger a seizure. Likewise, women who are pregnant should avoid internal, topical and aromatic use as well. For any individual, internal use of eucalyptus oil is discouraged, as it can be fatal in the wrong doses.

8.  **Frankincense:** Frankincense is very soothing, helping to alleviate anxiety and depression while promoting an overall increase in tranquility. If you ever find yourself in a period of extreme stress, add a few drops of frankincense oil to your bathwater and soak for twenty minutes while

visualizing all of your negative emotions melting away.  A few drops of frankincense oil on the pillowcase will ensure a restful night's sleep, while also increasing sexual energy.

On a physical level, frankincense is excellent at boosting the immune system, and can be used to keep all forms of sickness at bay! As the oil naturally repels germs, it is a popular natural remedy for alleviating dental issues, such as gum inflammation and gingivitis when mixed with water and used as a mouthwash

9.  **Ginger:** Ginger is one of the most versatile, valuable essential oils on the market today. It is powerful and stimulating in nature, meaning that it is wonderful for increasing the libido and overall

energy levels while promoting happiness,

confidence and an overall sense of self-

empowerment!

Ginger oil dramatically improves blood circulation

when incorporated into a bath or massage. However,

one of the most widely renowned properties of ginger

is its ability to soothe nausea and prevent motion

sickness. A few drops of the essential oil can be placed

on a cotton ball an inhaled for this effect, while a drop

or two in a mug of hot water will serve the same

purpose. While many pregnant women are able to

safely combat the effects of morning sickness by

drinking ginger tea or eating small amounts of candied

ginger root, it is vital to consult with a doctor before

consuming the oil internally if you are pregnant or

nursing.

10. **Jasmine:** Jasmine oil is highly beneficial for alleviating stress. Its calming fragrance eases anxiety and banishes depression, making this a highly effective treatment for those who battle with inner demons.  A few drops of the oil added to one's pillowcase helps to promote a restful sleep, while wearing the oil topically or adding it to the bathwater is said to assist with drawing romantic energy towards oneself while increasing the libido.

Jasmine oil is good for improving mild respiratory ailments. It is also highly effective at treating issues related to female menstruation, such as helping to alleviate cramping. Some midwives swear by diffusing jasmine oil throughout a room as a woman is giving birth to ease labor pains.  Although it is non-toxic and

one of the safer oils in general, women who are

pregnant or nursing should still avoid all forms of use.


11. **Lavender:** Lavender is perhaps the most popular

   essential oil in the world. It is widely renowned for

   its multitude of healing properties, both in regards

   to the mind and the body. Lavender is extremely

   soothing; therefore, it helps to promote a calm,

   tranquil environment. Diffusing lavender

   throughout a room will help to combat stress

   while promoting a general sense of well-being.

Lavender promotes restfulness; therefore, it is highly

effective in treating cases of insomnia. For children

who suffer from night terrors, a few drops of lavender

oil on the pillowcase will help to ensure a relief from

nightmares while promoting relaxation at the same

time. A few drops of the oil can be added to bathwater

or simply placed on a cotton ball and inhaled to guard

against migraine headaches as well.


Perhaps one of lavender's most valuable healing

properties is in regards to its amazing ability to treat

burns and scalds. A few drops of lavender oil applied to

the affected as soon as possible after burning helps to

not only reduce the pain and prevent against blistering,

it dramatically speeds up the healing process as well.

This healing quality is so marked that many people

keep a small bottle of lavender oil in their kitchen

specifically for this purpose!

12. **Lemon:** Lemon oil is uplifting by nature. The oil

helps to stabilize mood swings by promoting an

overall sense of happiness while increasing levels of vitality and energy. Lemon oil can also assist with improving concentration and maintaining focus.

Add a few drops of lemon oil to water for a powerful, all-natural cleaning agent that will fill your house with a delightful fragrance. Lemon oil is a natural anti-biotic, which means that it can help to prevent against disease and illnesses. Adding the oil to one's bathwater is a simple, easy way to boost the immune system, while diffusing the scent throughout the home helps to promote an overall sense of good health and well-being.

As with other citrus oils, lemon oil is extremely photosensitive. This means that you should never wear lemon oil if you are planning on spending any time in the sun. Even without exposure to sunlight, lemon oil can be very irritating to the skin, so be sure to use a quality carrier oil and conduct a spot test before applying in any sort of volume.

13. **Marjoram:** Marjoram oil is highly effective at alleviating anxiety while promoting a sense of calm and tranquility. If you are feeling overwhelmed by stress, adding a few drops of marjoram oil to your bathwater will quiet your mind almost instantly, making this a very effective remedy for over-excited children or those who suffer from mania, obsessive compulsive disorder, etc.

Medicinally, marjoram oil serves as a gentle digestive aid, helping to relieve constipation as well as soothing menstrual cramping. It can also help with alleviating mild respiratory issues and increases circulation when incorporated into massage.

**14. Patchouli:**  A grounding essential oil that is linked with stability and nature, patchouli oil is widely revered for its ability to increase the libido amongst both men and women. A particularly valuable essential oil for those who find themselves hindered by sexual inhibitions, diffusing patchouli throughout the bedroom or sprinkling it on the bedsheets helps to alleviate any negative baggage one may carry regarding sex, thus encouraging an enjoyable experience for both partners.

Patchouli oil is also excellent for treating a number of skin conditions. It repels bacteria, acts as an anti-fungal and discourages ticks, mosquitoes and other insects. While topical and aromatic use is generally considered safe, patchouli should not be taken internally, as there is no know safe dosage.

15. **Peppermint:** Peppermint is highly stimulating, being used to help increase energy and combat lethargy. Likewise, peppermint oil is valuable for boosting levels of creativity and concentration, as well as promoting an overall sense of mental alertness. Its energy is highly purifying, so it can be diffused throughout a room or area to remove any residual negative energy, or simply put a few drops in your bathwater after a long, stressful day

to remove any excess baggage that may be following you around.

Inhaling peppermint oil not only boosts energy levels, it can help to quell nausea and prevent motion sickness. Likewise, peppermint oil has been proven to alleviate migraine headaches while also carrying some mild respiratory benefits when applied to the chest. Peppermint oil is highly irritating to mice, spiders and ticks. Place a few cotton balls soaked in the oil in the corners of your home to guard against any unwelcome visitors or dilute the oil and use it on your clothing and backpack during hikes. It is important to note that peppermint oil is highly invigorating, thus it should not be used in any form less than five hours before you are planning on going to bed.

Peppermint oil can be diluted with water for its

analgesic and antibiotic effects as a mouthwash as well.

17. **Rose:** Just as jasmine oil is particularly beneficial for women, rose oil is the same. Not only does it help to alleviate feelings of stress, anxiety and depression, rose oil also helps to enhance beauty, attracts love and increases feelings of self-esteem. Diffusing the scent throughout a home is said to prevent against any sort of domestic arguments, while adding a few drops of the fragrance to one's bathwater is said to increase female sexuality and even promote fertility!

Rose oil can also be used as a powerful astringent and anti-acne tool. In fact, women are encouraged to mix three or four drops of rose water in with boiling hot water and hang their heads over the steam in order to

promote physical beauty and combat the external
signs of aging.

18. **Rosemary:** Rosemary oils is one of the most
powerful natural mental stimulants currently
available on the market. A simple whiff of
rosemary oil is invaluable in providing grounding
and stability while promoting wisdom and
increasing creativity. Students and professionals
alike can benefit from using rosemary oil to
improve levels of concentration and memory
retention while improving mental clarity.
Rosemary oil is showing promise in helping to preserve
the memory of patients with Alzheimer's disease. It
also has some pain-relieving effects when applied to
tired or sore muscles.

Rosemary oil should not be used in any form by pregnant or nursing women. It should also be avoided by anyone with epilepsy or other convulsive disorders, as well as people with hypertension.

19. **Sandalwood:** Sandalwood oil carries some very strong magical connotations with it. It is believed to assist with opening an avenue to the spiritual realms, promoting wisdom, assisting in acts of divination and promoting an overall strong sense of connection to the divine. For this reason, sandalwood oil is a particularly valuable addition to all sorts of religious and spiritual ceremonies, as it helps to establish a clear connection between the individual mind and the divine. Sandalwood is also heavily associated with sexuality and passion

as well. Particularly in regards to men, it restores virility and endurance while increasing levels of passion. Add a few drops of sandalwood oil to the bedsheets in order to loosen sexual inhibitions and encourage erotic play or wear the fragrance on the clothing to attract the attention of potential female suitors.

On a therapeutic level, sandalwood oil helps to relieve depressive symptoms as well as stabilizing the mood swings associated with premenstrual syndrome. Sandalwood also has sedative and calming properties, meaning that it can be used to promote a restful night's sleep as well.  Sandalwood oil can also assist with alleviating muscle tension and inflammation when applied topically. It reduces the severity and discoloration of bruises, and can also combat fungal infections, such as athlete's foot.

21. **Tea Tree:** Tea tree oil is one of the most valuable natural substances in existence. If you decide to work with only one essential oil, tea tree is the most beneficial choice. Not only does the aroma assist with improving mental function by encouraging clarity and boosting creative energies, the medicinal benefits are virtually unparalleled.

Tea tree oil is one of the most powerful topical anti-biotics and anti-fungal agents available. Not only does the oil kill germs on contact, it is a powerful repellent for biting insects, such as mosquitos and ticks. Tea tree oil is also a remarkable topical analgesic. It can be applied to fresh stings or bug bites for a numbing effect or use it on ingrown toenails to eliminate inflammation and infection while the nail is growing out.

# Quick Ailment Reference Guide

If you're ever stuck for which oil to use for which ailment, then just use this chapter as a reference.

**Alleviates Anxiety:** Angelica, bergamot, chamomile, frankincense, jasmine, lavender, marjoram and rose.

**Analgesic:** Tea Tree

**Anti-fungal:** Patchouli, Sandalwood and tea tree.

**Anti-inflammatory:** Sandalwood and tea tree.

**Astringent:** Rose

**Attracts Love:** Cinnamon, ginger, jasmine, rose and sandalwood.

**Boosts Creativity:** Angelica, cinnamon, peppermint and rosemary.

**Clarity:** Angelica, cedar, cinnamon, eucalyptus, rosemary and tea tree.

**Cleanses the Liver:** Bergamot

**Cleanses the Kidneys:** Sandalwood

**Cleanses the Spleen:** Bergamot

**Combats Depression:** Angelica, basil, bergamot, frankincense, ginger, jasmine, lavender, rose and sandalwood.

**Combats Migraines:** Angelica, basil, eucalyptus, lavender and peppermint.

**Cures Bruises:** Chamomile and Sandalwood.

**Dental Aid:** Frankincense and peppermint.

**Digestive Aid:** Ginger, marjoram and peppermint.

**Enhances Divination:** Sandalwood

**Febrifuge:** Eucalyptus

**Grounding:** Patchouli and rosemary.

**Heals Burns:** Lavender

**Improves Respiratory Function:** Angelica, cedar, eucalyptus, jasmine, marjoram and peppermint.

**Increases Appetite:** Basil and bergamot.

**Increases Circulation:** Cinnamon, ginger and marjoram.

**Increases Concentration:** Angelica, eucalyptus, lemon, rosemary and tea tree.

**Increases Confidence:** Cinnamon, ginger and rose.

**Increases Energy:** Angelica, basil, cinnamon, ginger, lemon and peppermint.

**Increases Sexuality:** Cinnamon, frankincense, ginger, jasmine, patchouli and sandalwood.

**Laxative:** Marjoram

**Memory Retention:** Rosemary

**Menstrual Aid:** Jasmine, marjoram and sandalwood.

**Natural Cleaning Agent:** Lemon and tea tree.

**Prevents Acne:** Chamomile and rose.

**Prevents Nightmares:** Chamomile and lavender.

**Promotes Good Luck:** Basil and cinnamon.

**Promotes Happiness:** Basil, bergamot, ginger, lavender and lemon.

**Prosperity:** Basil, chamomile and cinnamon.

**Protection:** Cedar

**Purification:** Cedar and peppermint.

**Relieves Nausea:** Basil, ginger and peppermint.

**Relieves Stress:** Bergamot, chamomile, frankincense, jasmine, lavender and marjoram.

**Repels Insects:** Chamomile, patchouli, peppermint and tea tree.

**Sleep Aid:** Chamomile, frankincense, jasmine, lavender and sandalwood.

**Spiritual Awareness:** Cedar and sandalwood.

**Stability:** Patchouli and rosemary.

**Strengthens the Immune System:** Cinnamon, frankincense, lemon and patchouli.

**Wisdom:** Cedar, rosemary and sandalwood.

# Creating Your Own Essential Oil Blends - DIY Recipes

Once you begin to experiment with essential oils, you may become tempted to begin creating your own specialized blends. One of the most important components in creating your own blends is to be sure you are storing them properly. You will need small glass bottles that are not tinted, as exposure to direct sunlight can alter the oil's compounds. Instead, elect for bottles that are dark blue or amber tinted in color.

From here, you want to fill each bottle with approximately two tablespoons of a quality carrier oil, the two best are almond oil and jojoba oil but you can also use apricot kernel oil. This is the base that you will use to construct any of the following recipes. It is important to store these mixtures in a cool, dry area, and be sure to shake them well before using. These essential blends rely on the concept of synergy. This means that one or more essential oils are combined due to their ability to work in harmony to treat a single need. In theory, their combined power is stronger than the single oil on its own.

Some of the most practical, popular essential oil recipes are as follows:

1.  **Anxiety Eliminator 1**

    3 drops jasmine

    3 drops rose

    3 drops frankincense

    Add to bathwater each night to promote restful

    sleep and relief from night-terrors or diffuse

    throughout the room for an overall sense of

    safety and well-being. Those who suffer from

    anxiety attacks may benefit from anointing

    their clothing with this blend or sprinkling it on

    their pillowcases and bedsheets.

2. **Anxiety Eliminator 2**

   2 drops bergamot

   2 drops marjoram

   3 drops lavender

   This is a wonderful concoction for eliminating a generalized sense of anxiety in both children and adults. It also assists with promoting happiness and promoting focus, which makes it particularly beneficial for anointing children's school bags and school clothes.

3. **Instant Calm**

   4 drops lavender

   2 drops angelica

   2 drops marjoram

This is an ideal blend for anyone who suffers

from panic attacks. Simply take a small whiff of

the blend for instant soothing, or use it in your

bathwater at night to prevent against a racing

mind or pointless worrying.


4.  **Nature's Antidepressant**

3 drops lavender

2 drops sandalwood

2 drops rose

2 drops bergamot

This is a wonderful oil blend for anyone who

suffers from depression, obsessive tendencies

or other mood disorders. It helps to promote a

gentle aura of happiness when diffused

throughout an area, or it can be worn on the clothing as a way of naturally uplifting the spirit.

5.  **Attracting Love**

2 drops jasmine

2 drops patchouli

2 drops sandalwood

1 drop cinnamon

Sprinkle amongst the bedsheet or diffuse throughout the bedroom to increase the libido while lowering inhibitions.

6.  **Happiness Blend**

2 drops bergamot

2 drops lemon

2 drops lavender

Diffuse through a room to promote an overall sense of joy and contentment.

### 7. Immunity Boost

2 drops lemon

2 drops eucalyptus

2 drops cinnamon

Diffuse throughout the household to promote overall good health.

### 8. Natural Insect Repellent

4 drops tea tree oil

4 drops patchouli

Mix with three cups of water and spray skin, clothing and bedding liberally to avoid ticks, mosquitos and other pests.

9.  **Natural Mouse/Spider Repellent**

4 drops peppermint oil

2 drops tea tree oil

Use the mixture to soak a cotton ball. Place one

cotton ball in all of the areas of the home to

discourage pests.


10. **Natural Sleep Aid**

2 drops chamomile

2 drops jasmine

2 drops sandalwood

Diffuse the mixture throughout a room or

sprinkle it onto bedsheets to ensure a good

night's sleep.

## 11. Nature's Housekeeper

4 drops lemon oil

4 drops tea tree

Place the blend in about two cups of water and mix in a spray bottle for an excellent, all-natural cleaning remedy that is non-toxic and safe for children and pets. Spray on kitchen counters, in the bathtub, toilet, sink or any other area to clean while preventing bacteria and germs.

## 12. Sweet Dreams

4 drops lavender

4 drops chamomile

2 drops jasmine

A simple whiff of this blend before bedtime

helps to promote restlessness or diffuse it

through the bedroom an hour before bedtime

to ensure that children receive a deep, pleasant

sleep.

## 13. Nature's Excedrin

4 drops lavender

2 drops peppermint

2 drops eucalyptus

The best way to use this formula is to simply inhale it at the first sign of a migraine onset. Even if you are not able to use it in the beginning phases, taking a small whiff every ten minutes or so will help to alleviate the worst of the symptoms. Those who are especially prone to stress migraines can combine two drops of lavender to the solution to help promote calmness as well.

**14. Nausea Relief**

3 drops ginger

3 drops peppermint

Inhale the scent directly from the bottle to alleviate the symptoms of motion sickness, or simply diffuse the mixture through a room to alleviate upset stomachs associated with morning sickness, hangover or digestive issues.

## 15. Passion Booster

3 drops cinnamon

2 drops rose

2 drops sandalwood

An ideal date-night blend, this is a wonderful addition to a couple's bath or massage, as it arouses the libido and promotes an aura of romance and sexuality. Sprinkle the mixture onto your bedsheet or clothes for the same effect or diffuse the scent throughout a room and watch the sparks fly!

## 16. Prosperity/Money Drawing Blend

3 drops chamomile

3 drops cinnamon

Use as a hand wash to increase monetary flow or use the oil blend to anoint the purse or wallet for the same purpose. The mixture can also be sprinkled around the house to promote overall good luck.

## 17. Protection

4 drops cedar oil

Use this mixture to anoint clothing to ward against accidents and other danger, particularly when traveling. This same mixture can be used on objects to prevent them from becoming damaged or stolen. When diffused in an area or sprinkled around the perimeter of a room, it guards against negative energies and wards off any malevolent entities that may be lurking nearby.

## 18. Bruise Remover

3 drops chamomile

3 drops sandalwood

Mix the oil blend with a cup of cold water and soak a rag in it to create a kind of compress. Drape the cloth over the bruised area for a few minutes to help improve discoloration and to discourage inflammation. Chamomile oil can be very irritating to the skin, so do not attempt this remedy unless you have used it topically before with no adverse effects.

## 19. Respiratory Aid

2 drops eucalyptus

2 drops peppermint

Mix with a quality carrier oil and rub on the chest for a decongestant effect or diffuse throughout the room or add to bathwater to aid with mild respiratory issues.

## 20. The Scholar's Blend

3 drops eucalyptus

3 drops lemon

2 drops rosemary

This is an excellent scent to diffuse throughout an area in order to enhance concentration and help with memory retention. Use it while studying or reading, then carry the bottle with you and take a deep breath of it before a test

or exam to boost focus and increase the ability

to recall what you have learned.


## 21. Stress Relief

2 drops jasmine

2 drops lavender

2 drops frankincense

Diffuse throughout a room or add to bathwater

to promote an environment of peacefulness,

calm and tranquility.

## 22. Woman's Best Friend

4 drops sandalwood

4 drops jasmine

Diffuse throughout a room or wear as a scent during one's menstrual period for obtaining relief from mood swings as well as to combat cramping and fatigue. This is also an excellent mixture to sprinkle upon the bedsheets to encourage fertility and increase female libido.

# Conclusion

And there we go, I hope you've enjoyed this book and that it's proved valuable to you. I urge you to try out some of the recipes listed as well.

One important thing to remember is to only buy high quality essential oils, sometimes cheaper brands pass off "massage oils" as being essential oils - but this is not the case. A surefire way to tell if an oil is fake is if they feel greasy or thick. The exception to this rule is sandalwood, which naturally has a thicker consistency.

Whatever your reason for using essential oils, they are a fantastic, natural way to remedy various ailments, both physical and mental.

Essential oils are quickly gaining recognition for their tremendous healing properties. There is absolutely no question that essential oils help treat the symptoms of different diseases as effectively or more than the drugs which are administered by pharmaceutical companies.

So best of luck to you in your essential oil journey - and I wish you all the best.

One final note, if this book has been useful to you - I'd really appreciate it if you left it a review on Amazon.

Thanks,

Lauren

## References

- **Bradford, Nikki** <u>Heal Yourself with Flowers and Other Essences</u> Quadrille Publishing, London, England, 2005.

- **Chapman, Judy** <u>Aromatherapy: Recipes for your Oil Burner</u> Harper Collins Publishers, Sydney, Australia, 1998.

- **Cunningham, Scott** <u>Magical Aromatherapy: The Power of Scent</u> Llewellyn Publications, Woodbury, Minnesota, 2006.

- **Dugan, Ellen** <u>Garden Witch's Herbal</u> Llewellyn Publications, Woodbury, Minnesota, 2009.

- **The Reader's Digest** <u>Magic and Medicine of Plants</u> The Reader's Digest Association, Inc. Pleasantville, New York, 1986.

- **Walji, Hasnain Ph.D.** <u>The Healing Power of Astrology</u> Prima Publishing, Rocklin, California 1996


- **<u>Online Sources</u>**

- Distilling Essential Oils: A Work of Art and Science

  http://doterra.com/US/en/brochures-living-magazines-winter-2013-2014-distilling-essential-oils

- Essential Oil Academy

  http://essentialoilsacademy.com/history

- Essential Oil Haven for Natural Health and Well-Being "<u>What Are Essential Oils?</u>"

  http://www.essentialoilhaven.com/what-are-essential-oils

- The History of Essential Oils

  http://www.healingscents.net/blogs/learn/186858
  59-history-of-essential-oils

- Most Popular Essential Oils

  http://aromatherapy.com/most_popular.html

- National Association for Holistic Aromatherapy

  "Exploring Aromatherapy"

  http://naha.org/explore-aromatherapy/about-
  aromatherapy/what-is-aromatherapy

- Taking Charge of Your Health and Well-Being "How

  do I Determine the Quality of Essential Oils?"

  http://www.takingcharge.csh.umn.edu/exploring-

  healing-practicies/aromatherapy/how-do-i-

  determine-quality-essential-oils

# Other books by Lauren Marshall

<u>Hemp Oil and CBD: Your Guide to Using Medicinal Oils for Physical Injuries, Mental Health & General Wellbeing</u>



<u>Hemp Oil and CBD: Your Guide to Using Medicinal Oils for Physical Injuries, Mental Health & General Wellbeing</u>